Homemade Healthy Dog Food

GUIDE + COLLECTION OF RECIPES

with delicious dishes and snacks to improve your dog's health and happiness.
Simple dishes for a healthy and joyful canine lifestyle.

-ALEX BENNETT-

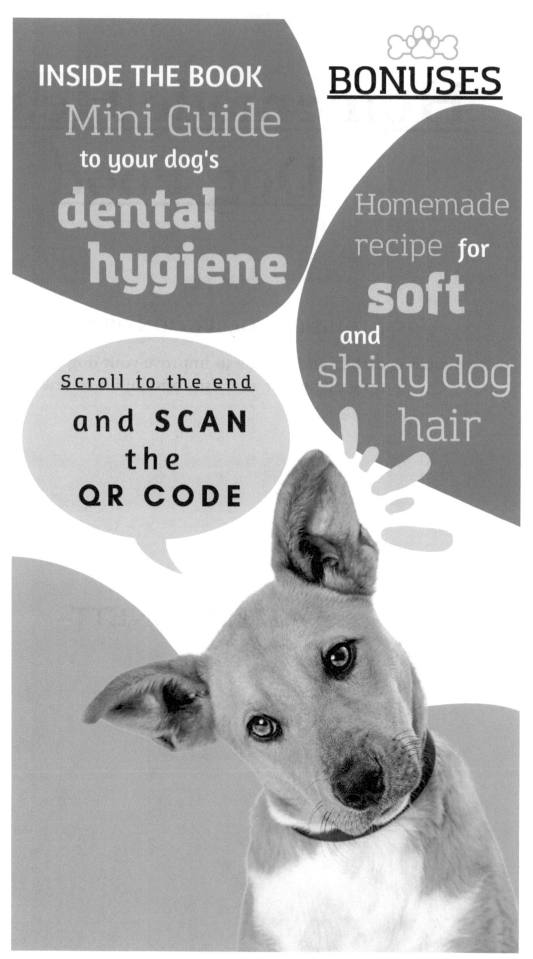

INSIDE THE BOOK

Mini Guide
to your dog's
dental
hygiene

BONUSES

Homemade
recipe **for**
soft
and
shiny dog
hair

Scroll to the end
and **SCAN**
the
QR CODE

Table of Contents

I. Introduction

A. Statement of Purpose

In the past few years, people have become more worried about the quality and ingredients of dog food sold in stores. As dog owners, we often wonder what's in the prepackaged food we buy for our dogs and if it's really good for their health and well-being. We think of our pets as members of our families, and just like we try to eat the best food for ourselves, we want the same for them.

This book, "Homemade Healthy Dog Food GUIDE + RECIPE COLLECTION filled with delightful meals and snacks to boost your dog's health and happiness. Simple, well-balanced, and pup-favored dishes for a vibrant, joyful canine lifestyle," has been carefully put together with a clear goal in mind: to help dog owners like you give your pets healthy, homemade meals that are tailored to their specific dietary needs.

The goal is not only to make sure your dog friend is in good health, but also to make them live longer so you can spend more time with them. You will find that this gives you a better sense of control over your pet's diet and helps you avoid possibly harmful ingredients that are often found in commercially made food.

This book will walk you through the complicated world of dog nutrition and help you understand which ingredients are safe and good for your dog and which ones you should avoid. It gives you an easy-to-follow plan for switching your pet from store-bought to home-cooked food, planning well-balanced meals, and making a variety of recipes that your dog will love.

This book has everything you need, whether you're busy and need quick and easy recipes or your dog has specific health needs that you need to take care of. It also gives cost analyses, so you know how to save money without sacrificing your dog's nutrients.

We talk about more than just feeding your dog. We also talk about keeping an eye on your dog's health and changing their food as needed. To make sure your dog does well on a homemade diet, you need to check his or her health regularly, know how to spot signs of food deficiencies, and make any necessary changes to the diet.

The journey to healthy dog food isn't just about making your dog live longer; it's also about improving the quality of the time you spend with your dog. Healthier pets are happier pets, and their joy and energy always affect our lives. With the information and tools this book gives you, you will be better able to make decisions about your pet's diet that will lead to a healthier and happy life for your beloved dog.

Let's go on this trip together to make sure our dogs have the best lives possible.

B. Benefits of Homemade Dog Food

Feeding our dogs a homemade diet comes with numerous benefits that extend beyond just the nutritional value. These benefits not only impact our pets' physical health but also their behavioral patterns and our peace of mind. Here are some of the compelling reasons to consider a homemade diet for your canine companion:

Tailored Nutrition: Every dog is unique, with its own set of dietary needs. A homemade diet gives you the opportunity to tailor your pet's meals to cater to these specific needs. You can account for factors like age, breed, weight, activity level, and health conditions, which is something that generic store-bought food often cannot provide.

Quality Control: When you feed your dog at home, you know exactly what's in their bowl. You can choose high-quality, whole food products and leave out the additives, preservatives, and fillers that are often found in commercial pet food. This amount of control can make a big difference in how nutritious your dog's diet is.

Diet Variation: With a homemade diet, you can offer a wider variety of foods to your pet. This not only makes meals more enjoyable for your dog but also ensures they're getting a broad spectrum of nutrients.

Allergy Management: If your dog suffers from food allergies or sensitivities, a homemade diet can be a lifesaver. You can easily eliminate problematic ingredients and experiment with different foods to identify what works best for your pet.

Improved Health and Longevity: A well-balanced, homemade diet can lead to observable improvements in your dog's health. This may include a shinier coat, healthier skin, leaner physique, higher energy levels, and better overall vitality. Over time, these health benefits can contribute to a longer, happier life for your pet.

Cost-Effective: While it may seem like making homemade dog food would be more expensive, it can actually be quite cost-effective, especially if you know how to shop smartly and make meals in bulk.

Strengthening Bond: Preparing meals for your dog can be a labor of love. It allows you to invest time and care into their well-being, which can deepen the bond between you and your pet.

In the following chapters, we'll explore each of these benefits in more detail, providing you with practical guidance on how to make a successful transition to homemade dog food. Remember, the goal here is not just to feed your dog, but to nourish them - and that's the significant difference homemade meals can make.

C. Brief Overview of the Book

"Homemade Healthy Dog Food: The Comprehensive Guide and Cookbook for Your Canine Friend" aims to provide you with everything you need to know about feeding your dog homemade meals, whether you're completely new to the concept or looking to improve and expand upon your current practices. Here's a brief overview of the content covered in this book:

Chapter 1: Understanding Your Dog's Nutritional Needs

We'll dive into the basics of canine nutrition to equip you with the knowledge necessary to provide a balanced diet for your pet.

Chapter 2: Ingredients to Include and Avoid in Your Dog's Diet
In this chapter, we identify safe and unsafe ingredients, helping you to make informed decisions when creating your dog's meal plans.

Chapter 3: Making the Transition from Store-Bought to Homemade Food
Transitioning your pet to a new diet must be done with care. We'll show you how to make sure your dog's move goes smoothly.

Chapter 4: Planning a Balanced Meal for Your Dog
You need to plan your meals if you want to eat well. This part tells you what vitamins and minerals your dog needs and how to give them to it.

Chapter 5: Quick and Easy Recipes for a Busy Week
We understand that time can be a limiting factor, so we have curated a list of quick and easy recipes that do not compromise on nutritional value.

Chapter 6: Special Recipes for Specific Health Needs
Whether your dog is overweight, has a heart condition, or is an active working dog, we provide specific recipes to cater to their needs.

Chapter 7: Batch Cooking and Meal Prep for Your Dog
Here, we introduce the concept of batch cooking and meal prep to help you save time while ensuring your dog always has a healthy meal available.

Chapter 8: A Cost Comparison of Homemade and Store-Bought Dog Food
This chapter will break down the costs of homemade meals compared to store-bought food to help you make an informed decision.

Chapter 9: Monitoring Your Dog's Health and Adjusting Their Diet Accordingly
Finally, we delve into how to monitor your pet's health, recognize signs of nutritional deficiencies, and adjust their diet accordingly.

In the appendices, you'll find additional resources such as sample weekly meal plans and the nutritional content of common ingredients.

By taking you on this journey step-by-step, this book aims to make the process of transitioning to homemade dog food as easy and seamless as possible. It's designed to give you all the tools, knowledge, and confidence you need to make this meaningful change in your pet's life. We believe that the love we share for our dogs is a powerful motivator to provide them with the best nutrition possible, and that is precisely what this book will help you to do.

II. Chapter 1: Understanding Your Dog's Nutritional Needs

A. Basic Nutrition Principles for Dogs

Understanding the basic rules of nutrition for dogs is the key to making a balanced homemade meal for them. Here, we'll break down the most important parts of your dog's diet and explain why each one is significant.

Protein: Dogs are mostly carnivores, but they can eat other things too. So, protein should make up a big part of their diet. Proteins provide important amino acids that are needed for growth, muscle development, tissue repair, immune function, and making hormones and enzymes. Meat, fish, eggs, and dairy are all great energy sources for dogs.

Fats: Fats are a dog's best source of focused energy. They give the dog needed fatty acids that its body can't make on its own. They also help the dog receive nutrients and are important for the way cells look and work.
The right kinds of fat, like omega-3 and omega-6 fatty acids, are also good for your dog's skin and body. Fish oil, flaxseed, chicken fat, and canola oil are all good sources of healthy fats for dogs.

Carbohydrates: Unlike people, dogs don't exactly need carbs in their diet, but they can still benefit from them. Carbohydrates can be a good source of fiber and energy. They can also help you digest food and keep your gut healthy. Carbs that are good for you can be found in whole grains, veggies, and some fruits.

Vitamins and minerals: The body needs these in small amounts, but they are important for a lot of different things. They help keep bones healthy, make hormones, keep nerves working, and do a lot of other things.
Many of the vitamins and minerals you need can be found in a healthy, well-balanced diet, but you may also need to take supplements.

Water: Staying hydrated is important for your dog's health because it helps with digestion, nutrient absorption, temperature regulation, and keeping all body processes going. Make sure your dog can always drink clean, fresh water.

When you cook for your dog at home, it's important to find the right mix of these items and make changes based on what your dog needs.
You also need to think about your dog's age, weight, breed, level of exercise, and health, as these can have a big impact on their dietary needs. It's best to talk to a vet or pet nutrition expert to make sure your dog's nutritional needs are being met.

In the next part, we'll talk about the different nutritional needs of dogs at different stages of their lives and those with certain health issues. This will help you further customize your dog's diet. By knowing these basic nutrition rules, you'll be well on your way to making tasty and healthy homemade meals for your dog.

B. Unique Nutritional Needs by Life Stage

Dogs, like people, have different food needs at different stages of their lives. Understanding these needs can help you give your dog a better food. Here, we'll talk about how your dog's nutritional needs change at different times of his or her life:

Puppies: Puppies grow and develop quickly, so they have high food needs. They need more protein and fat than adult dogs, and these nutrients should make up a big part of their food. The food a puppy eats should also have a lot of vitamins and minerals, like calcium and phosphorus, which are important for bone growth. Always feed dogs according to how big you expect them to get as adults. Small-breed puppies grow up faster and can be fed adult food before their larger-breed peers.

Adult Dogs: Once your dog hits adulthood, its nutritional needs will stabilize. The diet of an adult dog should be well-balanced, with a focus on keeping a healthy weight and supporting overall health. The food should include high-quality protein, carbs for energy, and enough vitamins and minerals. If they don't want to gain weight, the number of calories they eat should match how much they move.

Senior Dogs: As dogs get older, their metabolism slows down and their food needs change. Senior dogs usually need fewer calories because they aren't as active, but they still need a high-quality source of protein to keep their muscles strong. Diets for older dogs should also include omega-3 fatty acids to keep joints healthy and grain to keep the digestive system healthy.

Pregnant or Nursing Dogs: Pregnant and nursing dogs have increased nutritional needs to support the growth of puppies and milk production. They require more calories, protein, and certain vitamins and minerals. It's crucial to provide a balanced and nutrient-rich diet during this stage.

Dogs That Work or Are Very Active: Dogs that work or are very active have higher energy needs. Most of the time, they need a diet high in protein and fat to get enough energy and stay at a good weight.

Always remember that these rules can change based on the dog. Breed, size, health, level of exercise, and other factors can all affect nutritional needs.

When making a diet plan for your dog, it's a good idea to talk to a vet or a qualified pet nutritionist. This can help make sure that your furry friend gets the best nutrition at every stage of their life and lives a healthier, happy life. In the next part, we'll talk about what dogs with certain health conditions should eat.

C. Health Considerations and Diet

Just like people, dogs can have different health problems that can have a big effect on their food needs. Some health problems can be helped, at least in part, by making changes to your diet.
Here, we'll talk about some common health problems in dogs and how their food can be changed to support their health:

Obesity: Obesity is a common problem in dogs and can lead to many health problems, such as joint problems, diabetes, and heart disease. Dogs who are overweight or have weight problems should eat a diet that is low in fat and calories but high in fiber. This will help them feel better without giving them extra calories. Getting regular exercise and watching how much you eat are also important for weight management.

Allergies or food sensitivities: Dogs can be allergic or sensitive to certain foods, which can cause signs like itching, digestive problems, and skin problems. If your dog has a food allergy, the allergenic item needs to be found and taken out of the diet.

Gastrointestinal Problems: Dogs with digestive problems might benefit from a food that is easy to digest. This usually includes easy-to-digest proteins, certain types of fiber, and sometimes bacteria to help keep the gut healthy.

Kidney Disease: Dogs with kidney disease often need a diet low in protein and phosphorus. However, the protein they do consume should be of high quality. Always consult with a vet to properly manage kidney disease through diet.

Heart Disease: Canine heart disease often requires a diet low in sodium to prevent fluid buildup. Certain supplements like taurine and L-carnitine might also be beneficial, though you should always consult with a vet before adding supplements to your dog's diet.

Diabetes: Dogs with diabetes need food that can help keep their blood sugar levels in check. This usually includes eating a lot of fiber, which can slow the rate at which glucose enters the bloodstream. A consistent eating routine is also important for managing diabetes.

Arthritis: Dogs with arthritis may benefit from a diet high in omega-3 fatty acids, which can help lower inflammation. Some medicines, like glucosamine and chondroitin, can also support joint health.

Remember that if your dog has a health problem, you should always talk to a vet or pet nutrition expert before making any big changes to its food. Choosing the right food for your dog can make a huge difference in their health and quality of life.

In the next chapter, we'll talk about what ingredients are safe and what ingredients aren't safe for dogs. This will help you make smart choices when making homemade dog food.

III. Chapter 2: Ingredients to Include and Avoid in Your Dog's Diet

A. The Safe List: What Your Dog Can Eat

When making homemade meals for your dog, it's important to know what items are safe and good for their health. Here are some important things to include in your dog's diet:

Protein Sources: Lean foods like chicken, turkey, beef, and fish are great sources of protein for dogs. You can also include organ meats like liver and heart, which are full of important nutrients.

Fruits and vegetables: Many fruits and vegetables are safe and healthy for dogs. They can give you important vitamins, minerals, and fiber. Apples (without the seeds), bananas, blueberries, carrots, cucumbers, green beans, peas, sweet potatoes, and pumpkins are all great options.

Whole Grains: Whole grains like brown rice, quinoa, and oatmeal are good sources of carbohydrates and can give your dog slow-releasing energy.

Eggs and milk: Eggs are a great source of easily digested protein, riboflavin, and selenium. Some dogs can also eat dairy products like plain yogurt and cottage cheese, which can provide extra protein and calcium.

Healthy Fats: Healthy fats like fish oil, flaxseed oil, olive oil, and coconut oil contain essential fatty acids like Omega-3 and Omega-6, which are good for your dog's skin, coat, and general health.

Bone broth: Bone broth is a nutrient-dense liquid that can provide vitamins, help improve joint health, and support a healthy digestive system.

Remember to introduce new foods slowly and watch for any bad responses. Even safe foods can cause problems for some dogs, such as food allergies or intolerances. When in question, talk to your vet or a pet nutrition expert. They can give you advice based on your dog's individual needs and help you make a balanced and healthy diet.

In the next part, we'll talk about the things you shouldn't put in your dog's food, so that your pet stays safe as you explore the world of homemade dog food.

B. The Unsafe List: What Your Dog Can't Eat

While many things are fine for dogs to eat, there are some that are poisonous and should always be avoided. Here are some things you should never put in your dog's homemade meals:

Chocolate: Chocolate has theobromine, which is bad for dogs. It can make you vomit, have diarrhea, breathe quickly, have a fast heart rate, have seizures, and, in the worst cases, even kill you.

Grapes and raisins: These fruits are very bad for dogs and can lead to quick kidney failure.

Onions and garlic: These veggies can cause anemia in dogs by killing their red blood cells. This includes all kinds, like raw, cooked, powdered, or dried.

Xylitol: This artificial sweetener, found in many sugar-free foods, can cause a rapid insulin release in dogs, leading to hypoglycemia (low blood sugar), seizures, liver failure, or even death.

Avocado: Avocado contains persin, a substance that can cause diarrhea, vomiting, and heart congestion in dogs.

Alcohol: Alcohol can cause vomiting, diarrhea, decreased coordination, central nervous system depression, difficulty breathing, and even death in dogs.

Macadamia Nuts: These nuts can make dogs weak, sick, tremble, and get too hot.

Caffeine: Products with caffeine in them, like coffee or tea, can make dogs anxious, breathe quickly, have heart palpitations, shake their muscles, and even have seizures.

Raw Yeast Dough: If a dog eats raw dough, it can rise in its stomach, causing pain, bloating, and even major problems.

Some chemical Sweeteners and Food Additives: Besides xylitol, some chemical sweeteners, colorings, and food additives can be bad for dogs.

This list isn't complete, and there may be other things that are bad for dogs. Before giving your dog new things, you should always check with your vet first.

In the next part, we'll show you how to switch your dog from store-bought food to healthy meals you make at home. This is a very important step to make sure that your dog will accept it and be healthy generally.

C. Identifying Potential Allergens and How to Deal with Them

Dogs often have allergies or sensitivities to certain foods, which can make it hard to make fresh meals for them. Knowing how to find possible allergens and how to deal with them can make a big difference in how healthy and happy your dog is.

Find out what causes common allergies: Any food could cause an allergic response in a dog, but some foods are more likely to do so. These include meat, dairy, wheat, eggs, chicken, lamb, pork, rabbit, soy, and fish. Keep in mind that dogs generally have food allergies because of the protein source.

Symptoms of Food Allergies: Itching, ear infections, skin infections, diarrhea, and vomiting are all common symptoms of food allergies in dogs. If your dog has any of these signs, he or she may have a food allergy or sensitivity.

Diagnosis and Testing: If you think your dog has a food allergy, a veterinarian can do tests to prove this. The most accurate test is an elimination diet, in which the dog is fed a diet free of common allergens for a certain amount of time (usually 8–12 weeks), and then possible allergenic foods are added one at a time to find the cause.

Taking Care of Food Allergies: If a specific allergen is found, the best way to treat the allergy is to keep your dog from eating that food. This means that when you cook homemade meals, you'll have to choose items that don't contain the allergen. Many dogs with food allergies do well on a diet with new proteins (proteins they have never eaten before) or hydrolyzed proteins (proteins that have been broken down so they don't cause an allergic reaction).

Consult a Veterinarian or a Pet Nutritionist: Dealing with food allergies in dogs can be challenging, and each dog may react differently. It's always best to work closely with a vet or a pet nutritionist when dealing with potential food allergies.

Food allergies can be a source of discomfort for your dog and a concern for you, but they can be managed effectively. The key is to identify the allergen and create a balanced diet without that ingredient. In the next chapter, we will start the journey of making homemade dog food by explaining the transition process from commercial food to homemade meals.

IV. Chapter 3: Making the Transition from Store-Bought to Homemade Food

A. Gradual Transitioning

Transitioning your dog to a homemade diet should be a gradual process to avoid upsetting your pet's digestive system. Sudden changes in diet can lead to issues like vomiting, diarrhea, or loss of appetite. Here are the steps for a smooth transition:

Start Slow: Begin by replacing a small portion of your dog's current diet with homemade food. A general rule is to start with 10-25% homemade food and 75-90% of their current food.

Monitor Your Dog's Reaction: Keep a close eye on your dog's response to the new food. Look out for changes in their bowel movements, energy levels, weight, skin, and coat. If your dog shows signs of gastrointestinal upset, slow down the transition pace.

Increase Homemade Food Gradually: Over the course of 7-10 days, gradually increase the proportion of homemade food while decreasing the amount of their old diet. This transition period can be extended if your dog has a sensitive stomach or is prone to dietary upsets.

Reach 100% Homemade Food: Eventually, your dog's meals should consist entirely of a homemade diet. Keep monitoring your pet's health and consult a vet if you notice any adverse reactions.

Routine and Consistency: Dogs thrive on routine, so try to feed them the new diet at the same times each day.

Consultation with a Vet or Pet Nutritionist: It's a good idea to consult with a vet or a pet nutritionist during this transition. They can provide specific advice based on your dog's health status and nutritional needs.

Remember, every dog is different, and what works for one may not work for another. Be patient, and don't get discouraged if your dog seems unsure about the new food at first. Keep the transition slow and steady, and before you know it, your dog will be enjoying their new, healthier diet.

In the next section, we'll delve into creating a balanced homemade diet, detailing the essential components every meal should have.

B. Monitoring Your Dog's Health during the Transition

Transitioning your dog to a homemade diet is not just about changing the food in their bowl. It's crucial to monitor their health throughout the transition to ensure the new diet is agreeing with them. Here are some ways to keep an eye on your dog's health:

Weight: Regularly weigh your dog to ensure they are maintaining a healthy weight. Rapid weight loss or gain can indicate a problem and should prompt a consultation with a vet.

Energy Levels: Notice if your dog's energy level has changed. A good diet should support your dog's normal activity level. If your dog seems overly lethargic or, conversely, hyperactive, it may indicate that their dietary needs are not being met.

Coat and Skin: A healthy diet often results in a shiny coat and healthy skin. If you notice dullness, excessive shedding, or skin irritation, it might suggest a dietary imbalance or a food sensitivity.

Bowel Movements: Monitor your dog's poop. Changes in color, consistency, and frequency can provide insight into how well they are adjusting to the new diet. Diarrhea, constipation, or unusually colored poop should be reported to a vet.

Appetite: Monitor your dog's appetite. If your dog is leaving food behind or seems excessively hungry, it could indicate that you're not serving the right portion sizes or that the food isn't satisfying them.

Behavior Changes: Keep an eye on any changes in your dog's behavior. Agitation, excessive licking, or changes in sleeping patterns can sometimes be linked to diet changes.

Regular Vet Check-ups: Regular vet check-ups are crucial during the transition period. A professional can monitor your dog's health, conduct necessary tests, and confirm if the new diet is working well for your dog.

Remember, you know your dog best. If you notice any changes that concern you, don't hesitate to consult with a vet. The transition period is critical and will set the tone for your dog's experience with homemade food.

In the next chapter, we'll discuss how to ensure your homemade dog food is balanced and nutritionally adequate, which is vital for your dog's overall health.

C. Potential Challenges and How to Overcome Them

While transitioning your dog to a homemade diet can have numerous benefits, it's not without potential challenges. Here are some common issues you may face and ways to overcome them:

Picky Eaters: Some dogs may initially be hesitant to try homemade food, especially if they're used to commercial food. Overcoming this requires patience. Introduce new foods slowly and stick with it. You can also try warming the food slightly to release its aroma, making it more appealing to your dog.

Time and Convenience: Making homemade dog food can be time-consuming compared to buying ready-made food. To overcome this, consider making meals in bulk and freezing portions for later use. You can also invest in a slow cooker, which allows you to prepare meals with minimal hands-on time.

Cost: While some homemade meals may be cheaper than commercial dog food, others may be more expensive, depending on the ingredients. Research and planning can help keep costs down. Also, remember that investing in your dog's nutrition now can potentially save on vet bills in the future.

Ensuring a Balanced Diet: One of the biggest challenges of homemade dog food is ensuring that the meals are nutritionally balanced. Working with a vet or a pet nutritionist can help ensure that your recipes meet all of your dog's nutritional needs.

Food Safety: Just like human food, homemade dog food can be subject to spoilage and contamination. Ensure to store food properly and maintain good hygiene when preparing meals.

Health Concerns: If your dog has specific health conditions, a homemade diet may need to be tailored to their needs. Always consult with a vet if your dog has health issues before starting a homemade diet.

Remember, the key to overcoming these challenges is planning, patience, and seeking professional advice as needed. Making your dog's food at home can be a rewarding experience that enhances your bond with your pet while promoting better health.

In the upcoming chapters, we'll be getting into the fun part - recipes! We'll provide you with easy, nutritious, and delicious recipes to start you on your journey of homemade dog food.

V. Chapter 4: Planning a Balanced Meal for Your Dog

A. Portion Size and Caloric Needs

Portion size and caloric intake are two crucial aspects of feeding your dog. Serving the correct portions ensures your dog gets the right amount of nutrients without overeating, while understanding your dog's caloric needs helps maintain a healthy weight. Let's look at how to determine these:

Caloric Needs: Dogs, like people, have different caloric needs based on their age, size, breed, activity level, and health status. As a general rule, an average active adult dog needs about 30 calories per pound of body weight per day. Puppies and younger dogs usually require more, as do pregnant or lactating dogs. Older, less active dogs may need fewer calories. Consult with your vet or a pet nutritionist to determine your dog's exact caloric needs.

Portion Size: Once you know how many calories your dog needs, you can determine the correct portion size. Homemade dog food recipes should provide an approximate calorie count per serving. Divide your dog's total daily calories by the number of meals you feed them each day to find out how much they should eat per meal.

Monitor Weight: Regularly weigh your dog to ensure they are maintaining a healthy weight. If they start to gain or lose weight, adjust portion sizes or their total caloric intake accordingly.

Meal Frequency: Most dogs do well with two meals a day, but puppies usually require three to four meals. This can vary depending on your dog's specific needs.

Remember, every dog is different, and individual caloric needs can vary. Regular vet check-ups can help ensure that your dog's weight and overall health are on track.

In the next section, we'll dive into how to balance the main nutritional components in your dog's diet, including proteins, carbohydrates, and fats. We'll provide guidelines on what proportion of your dog's meal should be dedicated to each.

B. Balance of Protein, Carbs, and Fats

A balanced dog meal should have the right mix of proteins, carbohydrates, and fats. Each of these nutrients plays a vital role in your dog's health, but they need to be provided in the correct ratios. Let's break down each component:

Protein: Protein is essential for building and repairing tissues, and it provides the building blocks for enzymes, hormones, and antibodies. Dogs, especially puppies and active dogs, need a diet rich in high-quality proteins. Roughly 25-30% of your dog's meal should be made up of proteins. Good sources include lean meats, fish, eggs, and dairy.

Carbohydrates: Carbohydrates provide energy and are important for gut health. They should make up about 30-40% of your dog's meal. Choose complex carbs like sweet potatoes, brown rice, oats, or quinoa over simple carbs.

Fats: Fats are the most concentrated source of energy for dogs. They're essential for absorbing vitamins and protecting nerves, and they contribute to skin and coat health. Fats should make up about 25-30% of your dog's meal. Quality sources include fish oil, flaxseed, chia seeds, and meat fats.

Fruits and Vegetables: In addition to proteins, carbs, and fats, your dog's diet should include fruits and vegetables, which provide fiber, vitamins, and minerals. These should make up the remaining 10-20% of your dog's meal.

Remember, these percentages are general guidelines and may need to be adjusted based on your dog's specific needs. Consulting with a vet or a pet nutritionist can provide guidance tailored to your dog's age, breed, weight, activity level, and health status.

In the next section, we'll discuss the importance of adding supplements to your dog's homemade diet to ensure they're getting all the nutrients they need.

C. The Importance of Vitamins and Minerals

While proteins, carbohydrates, and fats are the main components of your dog's diet, vitamins and minerals play a critical role in maintaining their overall health. They are involved in numerous biological processes, including bone formation, hormone production, nerve function, and digestion. Let's delve into their importance:

Vitamins: Vitamins are essential for various metabolic reactions. For instance, vitamin A is crucial for vision, skin, and immune health. B vitamins support energy metabolism and nerve function. Vitamin D is necessary for bone health, while vitamin E acts as an antioxidant. Many of these vitamins are present in the foods you'll be serving your dog, but some may need to be supplemented, particularly if your dog has specific health issues.

Minerals: Minerals like calcium, phosphorus, potassium, and magnesium are vital for bone development, nerve transmission, fluid balance, and various other functions. Again, many of these will come from the food your dog eats, but others might need to be added separately. For example, dogs on a homemade diet often need a balanced calcium supplement to ensure they're getting the correct amount.

Supplementing Wisely: It's important to make sure your dog gets all the vitamins and minerals he needs, but it's also important not to give him too much, since too many vitamins and minerals can be dangerous. Always consult with your vet or a pet nutritionist before starting any supplementation regimen.

Quality Matters: When choosing supplements, opt for high-quality products from reputable manufacturers. Look for products that have been tested for purity and potency, and that are free from unnecessary fillers and additives.

Special Needs: Dogs with certain health conditions may require additional vitamins and minerals. For example, older dogs often benefit from supplements that support joint health, like glucosamine and chondroitin. Your vet can provide guidance based on your dog's individual needs.

Remember, every dog's nutritional requirements are unique, and their needs can change with age and health status. Regular check-ups with your vet can help you keep up with your dog's nutritional needs and make necessary adjustments to their diet.

In the next chapter, we'll start to explore a variety of delicious and nutritious homemade dog food recipes that your furry friend is sure to love!

VI. Chapter 5: Quick and Easy Recipes for a Busy Week

A. Breakfast Recipes

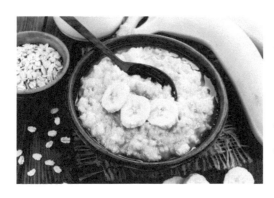

Peanut Butter and Banana Oats

Preparation Time: 10 minutes | Cooking Time: 15 minutes | Serving Size: 4 servings

Ingredients:
- 2 ripe bananas, mashed
- 1 cup of oats
- 1 cup of water
- 2 tablespoons of natural, unsalted peanut butter
- A pinch of cinnamon (optional)

Instructions:

In a medium-sized pot, bring the water to a boil.

Reduce the heat to medium and stir in the oats.

Cook the oats, stirring occasionally, for about 10 minutes or until the oats are tender and the water is absorbed.

Remove from heat and let it cool for a bit before adding the mashed bananas and peanut butter. Stir until well combined. If you choose to use cinnamon, add it now.

Allow the mixture to cool down before serving it to your dog.

Storage:

This dish can be stored in an airtight container in the refrigerator for up to 5 days. You can serve it cold or slightly warmed.

Nutrition Facts: Calories: 185 | Protein: 7g | Carbs: 25g | Fat: 7g | Fiber: 4g

Blueberry and Spinach Smoothie

Preparation Time: 5 minutes | Cooking Time: 0 minutes | Serving Size: 2 servings

Ingredients:

- 1 cup of spinach
- 1/2 cup of blueberries
- 1 ripe banana
- 1/2 cup of plain Greek yogurt
- 1/4 cup of water

Instructions:

Add all the ingredients (spinach, blueberries, banana, Greek yogurt, and water) to a blender.

Blend until smooth.

Serve in a dog-friendly dish, ensuring it is cool enough for your dog to consume.

Storage:

The leftover smoothie can be stored in the refrigerator in an airtight container for up to 24 hours.

Nutrition Facts: Calories: 80 | Protein: 5g | Carbs: 13g | Fat: 1g | Fiber: 2

Apple and Turkey Sausage

Preparation Time: 5 minutes | Cooking Time: 15 minutes | Serving Size: 1 serving

Ingredients:

- 1 turkey sausage
- 1/2 an apple, diced

Instructions:

Cook the turkey sausage in a pan over medium heat until fully cooked. This typically takes around 10-15 minutes.

Remove the sausage from the pan and let it cool.

Once cooled, dice the sausage into small, bite-sized pieces.

Mix the diced sausage with the diced apple.

Serve in a dog-friendly dish once it has cooled to a safe temperature.

Storage:

This dish can be stored in an airtight container in the refrigerator for up to 2 days.

Nutrition Facts: Calories: 140 | Protein: 10g | Carbs: 6g | Fat: 8g | Fiber: 1g

Sardine Scramble

Preparation Time: 5 minutes | Cooking Time: 10 minutes | Serving Size: 1 serving

Ingredients:

1 can of sardines in water, drained

1 egg

Instructions:

Heat a non-stick pan over medium heat.

Crack the egg into the pan and scramble it with a spatula.

Once the egg starts to set, add the drained sardines to the pan.

Continue cooking until the egg is fully cooked and the sardines are warmed through.

Allow the dish to cool to a safe temperature before serving it in a dog-friendly dish.

Storage:

This dish can be stored in an airtight container in the refrigerator for up to 1 day.

Nutrition Facts: Calories: 200 | Protein: 25g | Carbs: 1g | Fat: 10g | Fiber: 0g

Pumpkin and Quinoa Porridge

Preparation Time: 5 minutes | Cooking Time: 15 minutes | Serving Size: 2 servings

Ingredients:

- 1/2 cup of quinoa
- 1 cup of water
- 1/4 cup of pumpkin puree

Instructions:

Rinse the quinoa under cold water until the water runs clear.

In a saucepan, combine the rinsed quinoa with the water.

Bring the mixture to a boil over medium heat.

Once boiling, reduce the heat to low and cover the saucepan. Allow the quinoa to simmer for about 10-15 minutes, or until it becomes fluffy and all the water has been absorbed.

Remove the saucepan from the heat and let the quinoa cool.

Once cooled, mix in the pumpkin puree until well combined.

Serve the porridge in a dog-friendly dish at a safe temperature.

Storage:

This dish can be stored in an airtight container in the refrigerator for up to 3 days.

Nutrition Facts: Calories: 110 | Protein: 4g | Carbs: 20g | Fat: 2g | Fiber: 3g

Rice and Veggie Mix

Preparation Time: 5 minutes | Cooking Time: 20 minutes | Serving Size: 2 servings

Ingredients:

- 1/2 cup of cooked brown rice
- 1/4 cup of cooked peas
- 1/4 cup of cooked carrots (diced)

Instructions:

Cook the brown rice as per package instructions. Usually, this involves combining the rice with water in a 2:1 ratio and bringing it to a boil, then reducing the heat to low, covering, and letting it simmer until the water is absorbed and the rice is tender.

Meanwhile, steam or boil the peas and carrots until they are soft.

Once all components are cooked and cooled, combine the rice, peas, and carrots in a bowl and mix well.

Serve the mixture in a dog-friendly dish at a safe temperature.

Storage:

This dish can be stored in an airtight container in the refrigerator for up to 3 days. Warm slightly before serving again.

Nutrition Facts: Calories: 150 | Protein: 4g | Carbs: 32g | Fat: 1g | Fiber: 3g

Cottage Cheese and Fruit

Preparation Time: 10 minutes | No Cooking Time | Serving Size: 1-2 servings

Ingredients:

- 1/2 cup of cottage cheese
- 1/4 cup of diced strawberries
- 1/4 cup of diced blueberries

Instructions:

Wash and dice the strawberries and blueberries. Be sure to remove any stems or leaves.

In a bowl, combine the cottage cheese with the diced fruit.

Mix until the fruit is evenly distributed throughout the cottage cheese.

Serve in a dog-friendly dish at a safe temperature.

Storage:

This dish can be stored in an airtight container in the refrigerator for up to 2 days.

Nutrition Facts: Calories: 120 | Protein: 14g | Carbs: 10g | Fat: 2g | Fiber: 2g

Chicken and Sweet Potato Hash

Preparation Time: 15 minutes | Cooking Time: 20 minutes | Serving Size: 1-2 servings

Ingredients:

- 1/2 cup of shredded chicken (cooked)
- 1/2 cup of diced sweet potatoes
- 1/4 cup of diced green bell pepper

Instructions:

Dice the sweet potatoes and green bell pepper into small, bite-sized pieces.

In a non-stick pan over medium heat, cook the sweet potatoes and green bell pepper until they are soft, which should take about 10-15 minutes.

Add the shredded chicken to the pan and continue to cook for a few more minutes until the chicken is heated through.

Allow the dish to cool before serving to your dog.

Storage:

You can store any leftovers in an airtight container in the refrigerator for up to 3 days.

Note:

Always consult with your vet before introducing new foods to your dog's diet.

Nutrition Facts: Calories: 250 | Protein: 20g | Carbs: 18g | Fat: 10g | Fiber: 3g

Fish and Brown Rice

Preparation Time: 10 minutes | Cooking Time: 15 minutes | Serving Size: 1-2 servings

Ingredients:

- 1 small fillet of fish (like salmon or white fish)
- 1/2 cup of cooked brown rice

Instructions:

Rinse the fish fillet under cold water and pat it dry.

In a non-stick pan over medium heat, cook the fish until it flakes easily with a fork. This should take around 5-10 minutes depending on the thickness of the fillet.

Allow the fish to cool before flaking it into bite-sized pieces with a fork.

Combine the flaked fish and the cooked brown rice in a bowl. Mix well to evenly distribute the fish throughout the rice.

Allow the dish to cool before serving to your dog.

Storage:

You can store any leftovers in an airtight container in the refrigerator for up to 3 days.

Nutrition Facts: Calories: 220 | Protein: 18g | Carbs: 26g | Fat: 6g | Fiber: 2g

Yogurt and Mixed Berries

Preparation Time: 5 minutes | No Cooking | Serving Size: 1-2 servings

Ingredients:

- 1/2 cup of plain Greek yogurt
- 1/4 cup of mixed berries (like blueberries and strawberries)

Instructions:

Rinse the berries under cold water and pat dry.

In a bowl, combine the Greek yogurt and the mixed berries.

Mix them well until the berries are evenly distributed throughout the yogurt.

Serve immediately in your dog's bowl.

Storage:

It's recommended to serve this dish immediately after preparation. If there are leftovers, you can store it in an airtight container in the refrigerator for up to 24 hours.

Nutrition Facts: Calories: 110 | Protein: 10g | Carbs: 8g | Fat: 3g | Fiber: 1g

B. Dinner Recipes

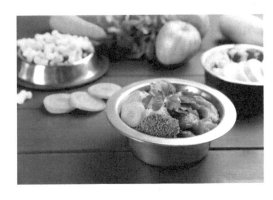

Lamb and Barley Bowl

Preparation Time: 10 minutes | Cooking Time: 15 minutes | Serving Size: 2-3 servings

Ingredients:
- 1/2 pound of ground lamb
- 1/2 cup of cooked barley
- 1/4 cup of diced zucchini
- 1/4 cup of diced carrots

Instructions:

Heat a pan over medium heat and add the ground lamb. Cook until no pink remains.

While the lamb is cooking, wash and dice the zucchini and carrots.

Once the lamb is cooked, add the cooked barley, diced zucchini, and diced carrots to the pan.

Stir well to mix all the ingredients.

Remove the pan from the heat and allow the mixture to cool before serving it to your dog.

Storage:

This dish can be stored in an airtight container in the refrigerator for up to 3 days. Always ensure to heat the stored food before serving it to your dog.

Nutrition Facts: Calories: 420 | Protein: 22g | Carbs: 28g | Fat: 24g | Fiber: 4g

Chicken Stew with Veggies

Preparation Time: 10 minutes | Cooking Time: 30 minutes | Serving Size: 2-3 servings

Ingredients:

- 1/2 pound of diced chicken breast
- 1/2 cup of peas
- 1/2 cup of diced carrots
- 1 cup of chicken broth

Instructions:

In a large pot, cook the diced chicken breast over medium heat until it's fully cooked.

Add the peas, carrots, and chicken broth to the pot.

Reduce the heat to low, cover the pot, and let it simmer for 15-20 minutes, until the vegetables are tender.

Once done, remove from heat and let it cool before serving to your dog.

Storage:

You can store the stew in an airtight container in the refrigerator for up to 3 days. Warm it up before serving.

Nutrition Facts: Calories: 300 | Protein: 32g | Carbs: 15g | Fat: 10g | Fiber: 4g

Turkey and Rice Mix

Preparation Time: 10 minutes | Cooking Time: 20 minutes | Serving Size: 2-3 servings

Ingredients:

- 1/2 pound of ground turkey
- 1/2 cup of cooked brown rice
- 1/4 cup of diced green beans
- 1/4 cup of diced pumpkin

Instructions:

In a large pan, cook the ground turkey over medium heat until fully cooked and no pink remains.

In a large bowl, mix the cooked turkey, cooked rice, diced green beans, and diced pumpkin until well combined.

Let the mix cool before serving to your dog.

Storage:

You can store this mix in an airtight container in the refrigerator for up to 3 days. Warm it up before serving.

Nutrition Facts: Calories: 280 | Protein: 28g | Carbs: 25g | Fat: 6g | Fiber: 2g

Fish and Sweet Potato

Preparation Time: 15 minutes | Cooking Time: 20 minutes | Serving Size: 2-3 servings

Ingredients:

- 1 fillet of white fish
- 1/2 cup of diced sweet potatoes
- 1/4 cup of diced spinach

Instructions:

Heat a pan over medium heat and cook the fish until it flakes easily with a fork. Set it aside to cool.

In a separate pot, bring water to a boil and add the sweet potatoes. Cook until they are soft and easily pierced with a fork. Drain and let them cool.

In a large bowl, combine the cooked fish, sweet potatoes, and diced spinach.

Storage:

You can store this mix in an airtight container in the refrigerator for up to 3 days. Warm it up before serving.

Nutrition Facts: Calories: 210 | Protein: 25g | Carbs: 20g | Fat: 3g | Fiber: 3g

Beef and Quinoa Dinner

Preparation Time: 15 minutes | Cooking Time: 20 minutes | Serving Size: 2-3 servings

Ingredients:

- 1/2 pound of lean ground beef
- 1/2 cup of quinoa (cooked)
- 1/4 cup of diced broccoli
- 1/4 cup of diced carrots

Instructions:

In a pan over medium heat, cook the ground beef until no pink remains. Be sure to break it up into small, bite-sized pieces.

In a separate pot, cook the quinoa as per package instructions. Let it cool.

In a large bowl, mix the cooked ground beef with the cooked quinoa, diced broccoli, and diced carrots. Stir well until combined.

Storage:

This meal can be stored in an airtight container in the refrigerator for up to 3 days. Reheat before serving to your dog.

Nutrition Facts: Calories: 320 | Protein: 30g | Carbs: 25g | Fat: 10g | Fiber: 4g

Liver and Brown Rice

Preparation Time: 15 minutes | Cooking Time: 20 minutes | Serving Size: 2-3 servings

Ingredients:

- 1/2 pound of chicken liver
- 1/2 cup of brown rice (cooked)
- 1/4 cup of peas
- 1/4 cup of diced carrots

Instructions:

Rinse the chicken livers under cold water and pat dry.

In a pan over medium heat, cook the chicken liver until it is no longer pink.

Cut into small, bite-sized pieces for easier consumption.

In a separate pot, cook the brown rice according to the package instructions.

Once everything is cooked and cooled, combine the chicken liver, brown rice, peas, and carrots in a large bowl and mix well.

Storage:

This meal can be stored in an airtight container in the refrigerator for up to 3 days. Reheat before serving to your dog.

Nutrition Facts: Calories: 350 | Protein: 28g | Carbs: 30g | Fat: 12g | Fiber: 3g

Venison and Sweet Potato Dinner

Preparation Time: 15 minutes | Cooking Time: 20 minutes | Serving Size: 2-3 servings

Ingredients:

- 1/2 pound of ground venison
- 1/2 cup of sweet potato (cooked)
- 1/4 cup of diced green beans

Instructions:

Start by rinsing the venison under cold water and then pat dry.

Cook the ground venison in a pan over medium heat until no pink remains.

In a separate pot, cook the sweet potato until it's tender. Allow it to cool and then mash it.

Once all ingredients are cooked and cooled, mix the venison, sweet potato, and green beans together in a bowl.

Storage:

You can store this meal in an airtight container in the refrigerator for up to 3 days. Make sure to reheat before serving to your dog.

Nutrition Facts: Calories: 320 | Protein: 30g | Carbs: 18g | Fat: 12g | Fiber: 3g

Salmon and Peas Dinner

Preparation Time: 10 minutes | Cooking Time: 20 minutes | Serving Size: 2 servings

Ingredients:

- 1 salmon fillet
- 1/2 cup of peas
- 1/2 cup of carrots (diced)

Instructions:

Start by rinsing the salmon fillet under cold water, pat dry.

Cook the salmon fillet in a non-stick pan over medium heat until it flakes easily with a fork. Let it cool down and then flake the salmon into small pieces.

In a separate pot, steam the peas and carrots until they are tender.

Once all ingredients are cooked and cooled, mix the flaked salmon, peas, and carrots together in a bowl.

Storage:

You can store this meal in an airtight container in the refrigerator for up to 3 days. Make sure to reheat before serving to your dog.

Nutrition Facts: Calories: 300 | Protein: 35g | Carbs: 15g | Fat: 10g | Fiber: 4g

Turkey and Vegetable Mix

Preparation Time: 10 minutes | Cooking Time: 20 minutes | Serving Size: 2 servings

Ingredients:

- 1/2 pound of ground turkey
- 1/4 cup of diced zucchini
- 1/4 cup of diced squash
- 1/4 cup of diced carrots

Instructions:

Cook the ground turkey in a pan over medium heat until no pink remains.

Add the diced zucchini, squash, and carrots to the pan and stir well.

Cook until the vegetables are tender. Make sure all the ingredients are well combined.

Storage:

You can store this meal in an airtight container in the refrigerator for up to 3 days. Make sure to reheat before serving to your pet.

Nutrition Facts: Calories: 280 | Protein: 30g | Carbs: 10g | Fat: 12g | Fiber: 3g

Pork and Apple Dinner

Preparation Time: 10 minutes | Cooking Time: 20 minutes | Serving Size: 2 servings

Ingredients:

- 1/2 pound of ground pork
- 1 apple, diced
- 1/4 cup of diced carrots
- 1/4 cup of peas

Instructions:

Cook the ground pork in a pan over medium heat until no pink remains.

Add the diced apple, carrots, and peas to the pan and stir well.

Cook until the vegetables are tender and the apple pieces are soft. Make sure all the ingredients are well combined.

Storage:

You can store this meal in an airtight container in the refrigerator for up to 3 days. Make sure to reheat before serving to your pet.

Nutrition Facts: Calories: 320 | Protein: 25g | Carbs: 20g | Fat: 15g | Fiber: 4g

Chicken and Vegetable Casserole

Preparation Time: 10 minutes | Cooking Time: 25 minutes | Serving Size: 2 servings

Ingredients:

- 1/2 pound of diced chicken breast
- 1/2 cup of diced potatoes
- 1/4 cup of diced carrots
- 1/4 cup of peas

Instructions:

Cook the diced chicken breast in a pan over medium heat until fully cooked.

In a separate pot, boil the diced potatoes until soft.

Once the potatoes are cooked, combine the chicken, potatoes, diced carrots, and peas in a bowl and mix well.

Storage:

You can store this meal in an airtight container in the refrigerator for up to 3 days. Make sure to reheat before serving to your pet.

Nutrition Facts: Calories: 300 | Protein: 30g | Carbs: 25g | Fat: 5g | Fiber: 4g

Rabbit and Barley Bowl

Preparation Time: 10 minutes | Cooking Time: 20 minutes | Serving Size: 2 servings

Ingredients:

- 1/2 pound of ground rabbit
- 1/2 cup of cooked barley
- 1/4 cup of diced zucchini
- 1/4 cup of diced carrots

Instructions:

Cook the ground rabbit in a pan over medium heat until fully cooked.

In a bowl, mix the cooked rabbit with the cooked barley, diced zucchini, and diced carrots until well combined.

Storage:

You can store this meal in an airtight container in the refrigerator for up to 3 days. Make sure to reheat before serving to your pet.

Nutrition Facts: Calories: 280 | Protein: 25g | Carbs: 35g | Fat: 5g | Fiber: 6g

C. Snacks and Treats

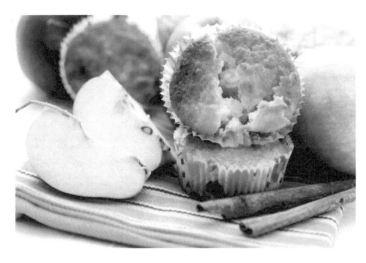

Carrot and Apple Pupcakes

Preparation Time: 10 minutes | Cooking Time: 15-20 minutes | Serving Size: Makes about 12 pupcakes

Ingredients:
- 1 apple (cored and grated)
- 1 carrot (grated)
- 1 cup of whole wheat flour
- 1/4 cup of oats
- 1/4 cup of apple sauce
- 1 egg

Instructions:

Preheat your oven to 350°F (175°C).

In a large bowl, mix together the grated apple, grated carrot, whole wheat flour, oats, apple sauce, and egg until well combined.

Scoop the mixture into a mini muffin tin, filling each cup about 2/3 of the way.

Bake in the preheated oven for 15-20 minutes, or until a toothpick inserted into the center comes out clean.

Allow the pupcakes to cool in the muffin tin for 10 minutes, then remove them to a wire rack to cool completely before serving.

Storage:

You can store these pupcakes in an airtight container in the refrigerator for up to a week, or in the freezer for up to three months. If frozen, thaw in the refrigerator before serving.

Nutrition Facts: Calories: 80 | Protein: 3g | Carbs: 15g | Fat: 1g | Fiber: 2g

Peanut Butter and Honey Dog Biscuits

Preparation Time: 15 minutes | Cooking Time: 30 minutes | Serving Size: Makes about 24 biscuits

Ingredients:
- 2 cups of whole wheat flour
- 1/2 cup of rolled oats
- 1/4 cup of dry milk
- 1/4 cup of cornmeal
- 1/2 cup of peanut butter
- 1/2 cup of water
- 1/2 cup of honey
- 1 egg

Instructions:

Preheat your oven to 350°F (175°C).

In a large bowl, combine the whole wheat flour, rolled oats, dry milk, and cornmeal.

Add the peanut butter, water, honey, and egg to the dry ingredients. Stir until well combined.

Knead the mixture until it forms a dough.

Roll out the dough on a floured surface until it's about 1/4 inch thick.

Use a cookie cutter to cut the dough into shapes and place the biscuits on a baking sheet.

Bake in the preheated oven for 30 minutes, or until the biscuits are golden brown.

Allow the biscuits to cool on the baking sheet before serving.

Storage:

You can store these biscuits in an airtight container at room temperature for up to a week, or in the freezer for up to three months. If frozen, thaw at room temperature before serving.

Nutrition Facts: Calories: 120 | Protein: 4g | Carbs: 18g | Fat: 5g | Fiber: 2g

Blueberry and Banana Dog Cookies

Preparation Time: 15 minutes | Cooking Time: 25 minutes | Serving Size: Makes about 24 cookies

Ingredients:
- 2 cups of whole wheat flour
- 1/2 cup of mashed bananas
- 1/2 cup of blueberries
- 1/2 cup of water

Instructions:

Preheat your oven to 350°F (175°C).

In a large bowl, combine the whole wheat flour, mashed bananas, blueberries, and water.

Mix until well combined, and a dough forms.

On a floured surface, roll out the dough until it's about 1/4 inch thick.

Use a cookie cutter to cut the dough into shapes and place them on a baking sheet.

Bake in the preheated oven for 25 minutes, or until the cookies are golden brown.

Allow the cookies to cool on the baking sheet before serving.

Storage:

You can store these cookies in an airtight container at room temperature for up to a week, or in the freezer for up to three months. If frozen, thaw at room temperature before serving.

Nutrition Facts: Calories: 80 | Protein: 3g | Carbs: 15g | Fat: 1g | Fiber: 2g

Quinoa and Pumpkin Dog Treats

Preparation Time: 20 minutes | Cooking Time: 20 minutes | Serving Size: Makes about 24 treats

Ingredients:

- 1/2 cup of cooked quinoa
- 1/2 cup of canned pumpkin (not pie filling)
- 2 cups of whole wheat flour
- 1 egg

Instructions:

Preheat your oven to 350°F (175°C).

In a large bowl, combine the cooked quinoa, canned pumpkin, whole wheat flour, and egg.

Mix until well combined and a dough forms.

On a floured surface, roll out the dough until it's about 1/4 inch thick.

Use a cookie cutter to cut the dough into shapes and place them on a baking sheet.

Bake in the preheated oven for 20 minutes, or until the treats are golden brown.

Allow the treats to cool on the baking sheet before serving.

Storage:

Store these treats in an airtight container at room temperature for up to one week, or in the freezer for up to three months. If frozen, thaw at room temperature before serving.

Nutrition Facts: Calories: 70 | Protein: 3g | Carbs: 12g | Fat: 1g | Fiber: 2g

Chicken and Carrot Dog Biscuits

Preparation Time: 20 minutes | Cooking Time: 20-25 minutes | Serving Size: Makes about 24 biscuits

Ingredients:
- 1/2 cup of shredded chicken
- 1/2 cup of grated carrots
- 2 cups of whole wheat flour
- 1/2 cup of rolled oats
- 1 egg

Instructions:

Preheat your oven to 350°F (175°C).

In a large bowl, combine the shredded chicken, grated carrots, whole wheat flour, rolled oats, and egg.

Mix until well combined and a dough forms.

On a floured surface, roll out the dough until it's about 1/4 inch thick.

Use a cookie cutter to cut the dough into shapes and place them on a baking sheet.

Bake in the preheated oven for 20-25 minutes, or until the biscuits are golden brown.

Allow the biscuits to cool on the baking sheet before serving.

Storage:

Store these biscuits in an airtight container at room temperature for up to one week, or in the freezer for up to three months. If frozen, thaw at room temperature before serving.

Nutrition Facts: Calories: 80 | Protein: 4g | Carbs: 13g | Fat: 1.5g | Fiber: 2g

Salmon and Sweet Potato Treats

Preparation Time: 20 minutes | Cooking Time: 20-25 minutes | Serving Size: Makes about 20 treats

Ingredients:

- 1 small cooked salmon fillet (deboned and flaked)
- 1/2 cup of cooked and mashed sweet potato
- 1 cup of whole wheat flour

Instructions:

Preheat your oven to 350°F (175°C).

In a large bowl, combine the flaked salmon, mashed sweet potato, and whole wheat flour.

Mix until well combined and a dough forms.

Roll the dough into small balls, about an inch in diameter, and place them on a baking sheet.

Bake in the preheated oven for 20-25 minutes, or until the treats are golden brown.

Allow the treats to cool on the baking sheet before serving.

Storage:

Store these treats in an airtight container at room temperature for up to one week, or in the refrigerator for up to two weeks. These treats can also be frozen for up to three months. If frozen, thaw at room temperature before serving.

Nutrition Facts: Calories: 70 | Protein: 3g | Carbs: 11g | Fat: 1g | Fiber: 1g

Beet and Cheese Dog Treats

Preparation Time: 20 minutes | Cooking Time: 20-25 minutes | Serving Size: Makes about 24 treats

Ingredients:

- 1/2 cup of cooked and grated beets
- 1/2 cup of grated cheese (cheddar is a good choice for dogs, but always confirm with your vet)
- 2 cups of whole wheat flour
- 1 egg

Instructions:

Preheat your oven to 350°F (175°C).

In a large bowl, mix together the grated beets, grated cheese, whole wheat flour, and egg.

Once the ingredients are well combined, knead the mixture until a dough forms.

Roll out the dough on a floured surface to about a quarter of an inch thick.

Use a cookie cutter to cut out the treats and place them on a baking sheet.

Bake in the preheated oven for 20-25 minutes or until the treats are golden brown.

Let the treats cool completely before serving to your dog.

Storage:

Store these treats in an airtight container at room temperature for up to a week, or in the refrigerator for up to two weeks. You can also freeze these treats and they will last for up to three months.

Nutrition Facts: Calories: 70 | Protein: 3g | Carbs: 11g | Fat: 2g | Fiber: 1g

Zucchini and Apple Bites

Preparation Time: 15 minutes | Cooking Time: 20-25 minutes | Serving Size: Makes about 24 bites

Ingredients:

- 1/2 cup of grated zucchini
- 1/2 cup of grated apple
- 2 cups of whole wheat flour
- 1 egg

Instructions:

Preheat your oven to 350°F (175°C).

In a large bowl, mix together the grated zucchini, grated apple, whole wheat flour, and egg until well combined.

Scoop the dough by spoonfuls and roll into small balls. Place the balls on a baking sheet.

Bake in the preheated oven for 20-25 minutes, or until the bites are golden brown and firm.

Allow the bites to cool before serving to your dog.

Storage:

Store these bites in an airtight container at room temperature for up to a week, or in the refrigerator for up to two weeks. They can also be frozen and will last for up to three months.

Note:

Always consult with a veterinarian before introducing new foods into your pet's diet.

Nutrition Facts: Calories: 70 | Protein: 3g | Carbs: 11g | Fat: 1.5g | Fiber: 1.5g

VII. Chapter 6: Special Recipes for Specific Health Needs

Low-Calorie Recipes for Overweight Dog

Maintaining a healthy weight is crucial for your dog's overall health. If your dog is overweight, it can lead to various health problems like heart disease, diabetes, and joint issues. Here are some low-calorie recipes designed to help manage your dog's weight without compromising on nutrition and taste:

Lean Chicken and Veggie Mix

Preparation Time: 15 minutes | Cooking Time: 20 minutes | Serving Size: Makes about 4 servings

Ingredients:

- 2 chicken breasts (skinless)
- 2 cups of mixed vegetables (broccoli, carrots, and peas)
- 1 cup of cooked quinoa

Instructions:

Fill a large pot with water and bring to a boil. Add the chicken breasts and boil until fully cooked, about 15-20 minutes.

While the chicken is cooking, steam the mixed vegetables until they are soft.

Once the chicken is cooked, remove from the pot, allow to cool, and then shred using two forks.

In a large bowl, mix together the shredded chicken, steamed vegetables, and cooked quinoa.

Allow the mixture to cool before serving to your dog.

Storage:

You can store this meal in an airtight container in the refrigerator for up to 3-4 days.

Nutrition Facts: Calories: 280 | Protein: 35g | Carbs: 20g | Fat: 5g | Fiber: 4g

Fish and Green Beans Dinner

Preparation Time: 10 minutes | Cooking Time: 20 minutes | Serving Size: Makes about 4 servings

Ingredients:

- 2 salmon fillets
- 2 cups of green beans
- 1 cup of cooked brown rice

Instructions:

Preheat your oven to 350°F (175°C).

Place the salmon fillets on a baking sheet lined with foil or parchment paper.

Bake for about 20 minutes or until the salmon is fully cooked and easily flakes with a fork.

While the salmon is baking, steam the green beans until they are soft.

Once the salmon is cooked, allow it to cool, then flake the salmon using a fork.

In a large bowl, mix together the flaked salmon, steamed green beans, and cooked brown rice.

Allow the mixture to cool before serving to your dog.

Storage:

You can store this meal in an airtight container in the refrigerator for up to 3-4 days.

Nutrition Facts: Calories: 310 | Protein: 28g | Carbs: 24g | Fat: 10g | Fiber: 4g

Turkey and Pumpkin Stew

Preparation Time: 10 minutes | Cooking Time: 25-30 minutes | Serving Size: Makes about 4 servings

Ingredients:

- 1 lb. ground turkey
- 2 cups of pumpkin puree
- 1 cup of peas
- 1 chopped carrot

Instructions:

Heat a large pan over medium heat.

Add the ground turkey to the pan and cook until fully browned and no pink remains.

Once the turkey is cooked, add the pumpkin puree, peas, and chopped carrot to the pan. Stir to combine.

Reduce heat to low and let the mixture simmer for 15–20 minutes.

Once cooked, remove the pan from heat and let the stew cool before serving to your dog.

Storage:

You can store this meal in an airtight container in the refrigerator for up to 3-4 days.

Nutrition Facts: Calories: 320 | Protein: 30g | Carbs: 22g | Fat: 12g | Fiber: 6g

Low-Fat Beef and Zucchini

Preparation Time: 15 minutes | Cooking Time: 30 minutes | Serving Size: 4 servings

Ingredients:

- 1 lb lean ground beef
- 2 zucchinis (chopped)
- 1 cup of cooked barley

Instructions:

Cook the ground beef in a pan over medium heat until it's fully cooked.

Add the chopped zucchinis to the pan and cook until they are soft.

Mix the cooked beef, zucchini, and barley together.

Allow the mixture to cool before serving to your dog.

Nutrition Facts per serving: Calories: 250 | Protein: 20g | Fat: 7g | Fiber: 4g | Carbs: 28g

Sweet Potato and Fish Mix

Preparation Time: 10 minutes | Cooking Time: 30 minutes | Serving Size: 4 servings

Ingredients:

- 2 white fish fillets
- 2 sweet potatoes
- 1 cup of peas

Instructions:

Preheat your oven to 350°F (175°C).

Bake the fish fillets for about 20 minutes, or until they are cooked through.

While the fish is baking, steam or boil the sweet potatoes until they are soft.

Once everything is cooked, mix the fish, sweet potatoes, and peas together.

Allow the mixture to cool before serving to your dog.

Nutrition Facts per serving: Calories: 275 | Protein: 22g | Fat: 6g | Fiber: 5g | Carbs: 35g

B. Low-Sodium Recipes for Dogs with Heart Conditions

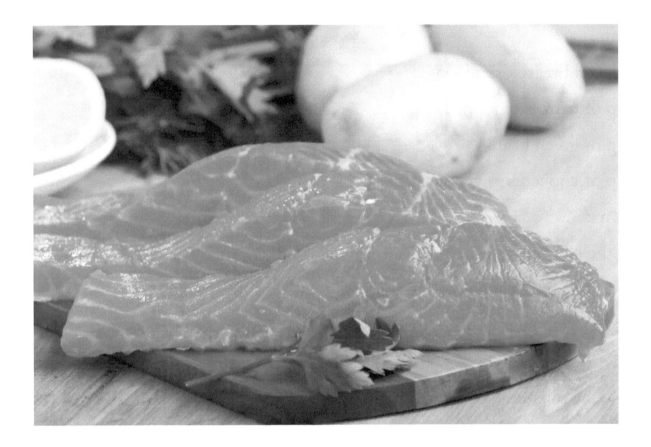

For dogs with heart conditions, a low-sodium diet is often recommended to help manage the symptoms and slow down the progression of the disease. Excess sodium can cause fluid accumulation in the body, which can strain the heart. Here are some low-sodium recipes that are both heart-healthy and delicious:

Heart-Healthy Chicken and Vegetables

Preparation Time: 10 minutes | Cooking Time: 30 minutes | Serving Size: 4 servings

Ingredients:

- 2 chicken breasts (skinless)
- 1 cup of carrots (chopped)
- 1 cup of green beans
- 1 cup of cooked brown rice

Instructions:

Boil the chicken breasts until they are fully cooked, then shred the meat.

Steam the carrots and green beans until they are soft.

Once everything is cooked, mix the shredded chicken, vegetables, and brown rice together.

Allow the mixture to cool before serving it to your dog.

Nutrition Facts per serving: Calories: 220 | Protein: 28g | Fat: 4g | Fiber: 4g | Carbs: 20g

Salmon and Sweet Potato Dinner

Preparation Time: 10 minutes | Cooking Time: 30 minutes | Serving Size: 4 servings

Ingredients:

- 2 salmon fillets
- 2 sweet potatoes
- 1 cup of peas

Instructions:

Preheat your oven to 350°F (175°C).

Place the salmon fillets on a baking sheet and bake for about 20 minutes.

While the salmon is baking, boil the sweet potatoes until they are soft.

Mix the cooked salmon, sweet potatoes, and peas together.

Allow the mixture to cool before serving it to your dog.

Nutrition Facts per serving: Calories: 240 | Protein: 26g | Fat: 6g | Fiber: 4g | Carbs: 24g

Turkey and Quinoa Meal

Preparation Time: 10 minutes | Cooking Time: 20 minutes | Serving Size: 4 servings

Ingredients:

- 1 lb ground turkey
- 1 cup of chopped zucchini
- 1 cup of chopped bell peppers
- 1 cup of cooked quinoa

Instructions:

Cook the ground turkey in a pan over medium heat until it's fully cooked.

Add the chopped zucchini and bell peppers to the pan and continue to cook until they are soft.

Combine the turkey, vegetables, and cooked quinoa in a large bowl.

Allow the mixture to cool before serving it to your dog.

Nutrition Facts per serving: Calories: 280 | Protein: 25g | Fat: 13g | Fiber: 4g | Carbs: 20g

Heart-Friendly Beef and Rice

Preparation Time: 10 minutes | Cooking Time: 20 minutes | Serving Size: 4 servings

Ingredients:

- 1 lb lean ground beef
- 1 cup of cooked brown rice
- 1 cup of steamed broccoli

Instructions:

Cook the ground beef in a pan over medium heat until it's fully cooked.

In a large bowl, combine the cooked beef, rice, and steamed broccoli.

Allow the mixture to cool before serving it to your dog.

Nutrition Facts per serving: Calories: 310 | Protein: 27g | Fat: 12g | Fiber: 2g | Carbs: 23g

Low-Sodium Veggie and Fish Mix

Preparation Time: 15 minutes | Cooking Time: 25 minutes | Serving Size: 4 servings

Ingredients:

- 2 white fish fillets
- 1 cup of chopped carrots
- 1 cup of peas
- 1 cup of cooked barley

Instructions:

Preheat the oven to 350°F (175°C).

Bake the fish fillets for about 20 minutes or until the fish is easily flaked with a fork.

In the meantime, steam the carrots and peas until they are soft but still retain some bite.

Once the fish and vegetables are cooked, mix them with the cooked barley.

Let the mix cool down before serving it to your dog.

Nutrition Facts per serving: Calories: 280 | Protein: 25g | Fat: 5g | Fiber: 6g | Carbs: 30g

C. High-Protein Recipes for Active and Working Dogs

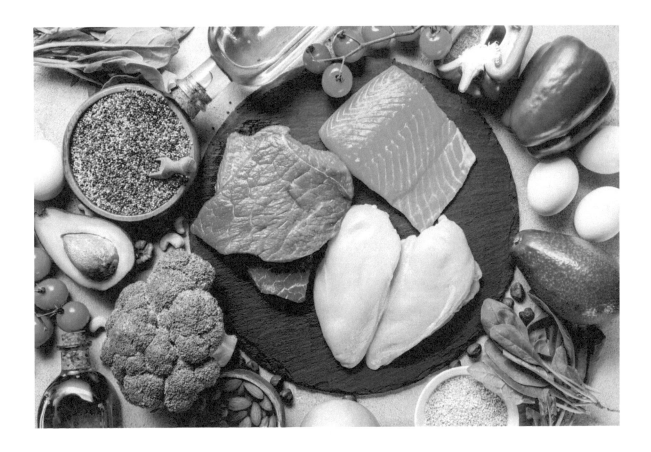

Active and working dogs require more protein in their diet to support muscle repair and growth, provide energy, and maintain a healthy immune system. Here are some high-protein recipes that are designed to fuel your dog's active lifestyle:

Active Dog Chicken and Quinoa Bowl

Preparation Time: 15 minutes | Cooking Time: 30 minutes | Serving Size: 4 servings

Ingredients:

- 2 skinless chicken breasts
- 1 cup of cooked quinoa
- 1 cup of cooked and mashed sweet potato
- 1 cup of steamed spinach

Instructions:

Boil the chicken breasts in a pot of water until they're fully cooked, usually around 20-25 minutes.

Once cooked, shred the chicken and set it aside.

In a large bowl, combine the shredded chicken, cooked quinoa, mashed sweet potato, and steamed spinach.

Mix everything until well combined.

Let the mixture cool before serving to your dog.

Nutrition Facts per serving: Calories: 300 | Protein: 28g | Fat: 6g | Fiber: 4g | Carbs: 35g

Turkey and Brown Rice Power Meal

Preparation Time: 15 minutes | Cooking Time: 20 minutes | Serving Size: 4 servings

Ingredients:

- 1 lb ground turkey
- 1 cup of cooked brown rice
- 1 cup of steamed broccoli
- 1/2 cup of cottage cheese

Instructions:

Cook the ground turkey in a pan over medium heat until it's fully cooked and no longer pink. This usually takes about 10 minutes.

In a large bowl, combine the cooked turkey, cooked brown rice, steamed broccoli, and cottage cheese.

Mix everything together until it's well combined.

Let the mixture cool before serving to your dog.

Nutrition Facts per serving: Calories: 325 | Protein: 30g | Fat: 12g | Fiber: 3g | Carbs: 25g

Beef and Vegetable Protein Mix

Preparation Time: 15 minutes | Cooking Time: 20 minutes | Serving Size: 4 servings

Ingredients:

- 1 lb lean ground beef
- 1 cup of cooked lentils
- 1 cup of steamed carrots
- 1/2 cup of peas

Instructions:

Cook the ground beef in a pan over medium heat until it's fully cooked and no longer pink. This usually takes about 10 minutes.

In a large bowl, combine the cooked beef, cooked lentils, steamed carrots, and peas.

Mix everything together until it's well combined.

Let the mixture cool before serving to your dog.

Nutrition Facts per serving: Calories: 360 | Protein: 35g | Fat: 10g | Fiber: 9g | Carbs: 30g

Salmon and Sweet Potato High-Protein Dinner

Preparation Time: 15 minutes | Cooking Time: 30 minutes | Serving Size: 4 servings

Ingredients:

- 2 salmon fillets
- 2 sweet potatoes (cooked and mashed)
- 1 cup of green beans (steamed)
- 1 cup of cooked quinoa

Instructions:

Preheat your oven to 350°F (175°C). Place the salmon filets on a baking sheet and bake for about 20 minutes, or until the fish is cooked through and flakes easily with a fork.

In a large bowl, combine the cooked salmon, mashed sweet potatoes, steamed green beans, and cooked quinoa. Mix well until all the ingredients are evenly distributed.

Allow the mixture to cool before serving it to your dog.

Nutrition Facts per serving: Calories: 450 | Protein: 37g | Fat: 15g | Fiber: 8g | Carbs: 40g

Egg and Chicken Active Dog Breakfast

Preparation Time: 15 minutes | Cooking Time: 20 minutes | Serving Size: 4 servings

Ingredients:

- 2 boiled eggs (chopped)
- 2 chicken breasts (boiled and shredded)
- 1 cup of cooked oats
- 1/2 cup of blueberries

Instructions:

Start by boiling your eggs. Once done, peel and chop them into bite-sized pieces.

Boil the chicken breasts until fully cooked. After they're cool to the touch, shred them.

In a large bowl, combine the chopped boiled eggs, shredded chicken, cooked oats, and blueberries. Mix well until all the ingredients are evenly distributed. Allow the mixture to cool before serving it to your dog.

Nutrition Facts per serving: Calories: 320 | Protein: 25g | Fat: 8g | Fiber: 5g | Carbs: 35g

VIII. Chapter 7: Batch Cooking and Meal Prep for Your Dog

A. Planning and Preparing Meals in Advance

One of the common concerns when switching to homemade dog food is the amount of time and effort it might take. But with a little organization and planning, you can ensure your dog has healthy, homemade meals every day without having to cook from scratch daily. Here's a guide to help you plan and prepare your dog's meals in advance:

Weekly Meal Planning:

Start by determining the number of meals your dog will need for the week. This will depend on their size, age, and activity level. Create a meal plan that includes a variety of proteins, carbohydrates, and veggies for balanced nutrition.

Recipe Rotation:

To prevent nutrient deficiencies and keep meals exciting for your dog, it's important to rotate the recipes you use. This doesn't mean you need to make a different recipe every meal. Instead, try to rotate them weekly or bi-weekly.

Grocery Shopping:

Once you have your meal plan and recipes, make a grocery list of all the ingredients you'll need for the week.

Buying in bulk can save money, but be mindful of the perishability of fresh ingredients.

Meal Preparation:

Choose a day of the week when you have a few hours to dedicate to meal prep. Cook all your proteins, grains, and veggies. Once everything is cooked, assemble the meals according to your recipes.

Portioning:

Use your vet's recommendation to determine the right portion size for your dog. Once the meals are prepared, divide them into these daily serving sizes. This step is crucial to ensure your dog isn't overeating or undereating.

Storing:

Once portioned, meals should be stored in airtight containers. You can refrigerate meals that will be used within the next three days. The rest should be frozen to preserve freshness. Thaw overnight in the refrigerator as needed.

Remember, while it might take a little extra effort initially, meal prepping can save you a lot of time during the week. Plus, it ensures your furry friend is eating a varied, balanced diet that's tailored to their specific needs. It's a win-win!

B. Storage and Shelf-Life of Homemade Dog Food

Understanding the best methods for storing and the estimated shelf-life of your homemade dog food is essential to maintain its freshness and nutritional value. Here's what you need to know:

Refrigerating Homemade Dog Food:

Once you have prepared your dog's meals, you should refrigerate them as soon as possible. If stored properly in an airtight container, most homemade dog meals can last for up to 3-5 days in the refrigerator.

Freezing Homemade Dog Food:

For longer storage, freezing is an excellent option. Portioned meals can be frozen in individual airtight containers or freezer bags. Frozen homemade dog food can last for about 2-3 months. Be sure to label each container or bag with the date to keep track of the storage time.

Thawing Frozen Meals:

When you're ready to use the frozen meals, transfer them to the refrigerator for thawing. It usually takes about 24 hours to fully thaw a frozen meal in the refrigerator. Once thawed, aim to use it within 48 hours. Avoid thawing meals at room temperature, as it can encourage bacterial growth.

Warming the Meals:

While not necessary, some dogs may prefer their food warm. You can warm the meal in the microwave or on the stove.
Be sure to mix it thoroughly and test the temperature before serving to prevent any hot spots that could burn your dog's mouth.

Discard Leftovers:

If your dog doesn't finish their meal, discard any leftovers after 2 hours if left at room temperature to avoid bacterial growth.

Remember, the key to safely storing homemade dog food is to keep it cold and airtight. If you notice any signs of spoilage such as an off smell, mold, or discoloration, discard the food immediately. When in doubt, it's always safer to throw it out. By following these guidelines, you can ensure your dog is eating fresh, nutritious meals every time.

C. Time-Saving Tips and Strategies

Incorporating homemade meals into your dog's diet doesn't have to be time-consuming. With the right strategies, you can streamline the process and make it manageable even on a busy schedule. Here are some tips to save you time and effort:

Batch Cooking:
Cooking in large quantities can save you a lot of time. Choose a day when you have some free time and cook for the week, or even the month. You can prepare different recipes and then freeze them in individual portions.

Use Slow Cookers or Instant Pots:
These kitchen appliances can be real time-savers.
You can put all the ingredients in the pot, set it, and go about your day. By the time you're done with your tasks, the dog food will be ready.

Pre-cut Vegetables:
Many grocery stores sell pre-cut veggies. While they might be slightly more expensive, they can save you a lot of prep time.

Utilize Leftovers:

Leftovers from your meals can often be incorporated into your dog's meals, given they are safe and healthy for them.

Just be sure to avoid any ingredients that are toxic to dogs.

Pre-Measure Ingredients:

When preparing meals, pre-measure all the ingredients and have them ready. This will save you time during cooking.

Rotate Recipes:

Having a variety of recipes will not only give your dog a diversified diet but also make meal prep less tedious for you. Rotate between recipes to keep things interesting.

Create a Dedicated Space in Your Freezer:

If you're freezing meals, have a dedicated space in your freezer. This will make it easier to store and locate the meals.

Invest in Quality Storage Containers:

Having quality airtight containers in different sizes can make storing and thawing meals much easier. Opt for stackable designs to save space.

Remember, the goal is to make feeding your dog homemade meals a sustainable practice, so find strategies and methods that work best for you and your schedule. By being strategic and using these time-saving tips, you can ensure that your dog benefits from a homemade diet without you feeling overwhelmed.

IX. Chapter 8: Cost Analysis: Homemade vs Store-Bought Dog Food

A. Price Comparison

Switching to homemade dog food is not only a nutritional decision but also a financial one. It's essential to understand the price comparison between store-bought dog food and homemade meals to determine if this change is feasible for your household.

Cost of Store-Bought Dog Food:
The price of store-bought dog food can vary widely based on the quality, brand, and type of food (dry, wet, raw, etc.). On average, you might spend anywhere from $20 to $60 per month for a mid-range brand for a medium-sized dog.

Cost of Homemade Dog Food:
The cost of homemade dog food also varies, depending on the ingredients you use. If you are using higher-end, organic ingredients, the cost might be on the higher side. However, it's possible to create nutritious meals with budget-friendly ingredients as well. On average, homemade meals might cost about $1 to $2 per pound, depending on the recipe. For a medium-sized dog, this could come to roughly $30 to $60 per month, assuming a daily intake of 1 to 2 pounds.

Consideration of Time and Effort:
While it's essential to consider the monetary cost, don't forget the time and effort required to prepare homemade meals. While some owners might find this task enjoyable and rewarding, others might find it challenging to fit it into their schedule.

Long-term Health Costs:
Investing in quality food can potentially save on veterinary bills in the long run. Dogs on a balanced, homemade diet may have fewer health issues, which could mean less spent on vet visits, medications, and special therapeutic diets.

Remember, these are average costs, and actual expenses can vary based on several factors, including where you live, where you shop, and any specific dietary needs your dog might have. It's always a good idea to do a cost analysis based on your dog's specific requirements and your local prices to get a more accurate understanding.

Switching to homemade dog food is not necessarily a cheaper option, but for many dog owners, the benefits of quality control, improved health, and the joy of providing for their pet's nutritional needs outweigh the costs.

B. Long-Term Savings and Benefits

While the immediate financial impact of switching to homemade dog food can vary, the long-term savings and benefits can be substantial. Let's look at a few key areas where these benefits can be seen:

Potential Health Savings:
One of the primary benefits of homemade dog food is the potential for improved health. A diet tailored to your dog's specific needs, using quality ingredients, can lead to fewer health issues. This could translate into savings on vet bills, medications, and special diets in the long run.

Quality of Life and Lifespan:
A balanced and nutritious diet can contribute significantly to your dog's overall quality of life and potentially extend their lifespan. While these benefits might not translate into monetary savings, they are priceless for any dog owner.

Avoiding Costly Recalls:
Commercial pet foods are occasionally recalled due to issues such as contamination. These recalls can result in unexpected costs, from replacing the recalled food to potential vet bills if your pet falls ill. Homemade meals help you avoid this risk.

Cost Efficiency with Bulk Buying and Seasonal Shopping:
Homemade dog food allows for cost savings through bulk purchasing and seasonal shopping. Buying ingredients in large quantities often reduces the cost per unit, and shopping for fruits and vegetables in season can also save money.

Reduced Waste:
With homemade dog food, you can prepare meals in the exact portion sizes your dog needs, reducing the amount of wasted food. Plus, it allows for using leftovers from your meals, given they meet your dog's dietary needs.

Control Over Ingredients:
While not a direct monetary saving, having control over what goes into your dog's meals can be considered a significant benefit.

You can ensure that your dog is eating high-quality, fresh, and wholesome food, free from preservatives, fillers, and additives found in many commercial foods.

In conclusion, while the cost of homemade dog food might be slightly higher or comparable to commercial food, the potential long-term savings and benefits make it a worthwhile investment. A healthier diet can lead to a happier dog and potentially lower veterinary costs, all while giving you peace of mind.

C. Budget-Friendly Tips for Making Homemade Dog Food

Making homemade dog food doesn't have to break the bank. With a few smart strategies, you can provide your furry friend with nutritious, homemade meals even on a budget. Here are some tips:

Buy in Bulk:

Purchasing ingredients in large quantities usually results in a lower cost per unit. Foods like rice, potatoes, and certain cuts of meat can often be purchased in bulk for less.

Shop Seasonally:

Fruits and vegetables are usually cheaper when they're in season. Plus, they're at their peak freshness and nutritional value.

Use Budget-Friendly Ingredients:

Some ingredients like lentils, brown rice, and certain vegetables are nutritious yet inexpensive. Incorporate these into your dog's diet to save on costs.

Consider Less Expensive Cuts of Meat:

Less expensive cuts of meat, like chicken thighs or ground turkey, are often just as nutritious as the more expensive ones. Organ meats, like liver and heart, are also less costly and are packed with nutrients.

Meal Prep in Bulk:

Cooking several meals at once saves time and energy costs. You can freeze the extra meals for later use.

Grow Your Own:

If you have the space, consider growing your own fruits and vegetables. This can be a fun and rewarding way to save money on ingredients.

Utilize Leftovers:

Provided they're safe and healthy for your dog, incorporating leftovers from your meals can be a great way to reduce waste and save on costs.

Shop Sales and Discounts:

Keep an eye on sales and discounts at your local grocery stores. Buying and freezing extra during these times can lead to significant savings.

Remember, the goal is to provide your dog with a balanced, nutritious diet. Always consult your vet or a canine nutrition expert when making significant changes to your dog's diet, especially when budget constraints are a concern. A homemade diet can be a great way to ensure your dog's nutritional needs are met, and with these budget-friendly tips, it doesn't have to be a strain on your wallet.

X. Chapter 9: Monitoring Your Dog's Health and Adjusting Their Diet Accordingly

A. Regular Vet Check-ups and Diet Adjustments

Despite providing your dog with the most nutritious homemade food, regular vet check-ups are crucial for your dog's overall well-being. They are important for several reasons:

Monitoring Weight and Growth:

Regular check-ups will help your vet monitor your dog's weight and growth. If your dog is gaining too much weight, your vet may suggest modifying the diet or increasing exercise. Similarly, if your dog isn't gaining enough weight, the diet may need to be adjusted.

Detecting Health Issues Early:

Routine check-ups can help detect health issues early, even before noticeable symptoms appear. Early detection often allows for more effective treatment and better outcomes.

Dental Health Check:

Vets also examine your dog's teeth during check-ups. Good dental health is vital for your dog's overall health.

Updating Vaccinations:

Regular vet visits ensure that your dog's vaccinations are up-to-date, protecting them from various diseases.

Nutritional Assessment:

One of the most important reasons for regular vet check-ups when feeding homemade meals is to assess whether your dog's diet is meeting all their nutritional needs. The vet might suggest diet adjustments based on your dog's age, weight, health condition, and activity level.

Even with the most carefully planned homemade diet, dogs' nutritional needs can change due to various factors like age, health status, and activity level. Regular vet visits allow you to make timely adjustments to their diet based on professional advice.

Remember, your vet is your partner in your dog's health. Keep them informed about any changes you observe in your dog's behavior, appetite, or physical condition. And be open about the diet you're providing so they can give you the best advice tailored to your dog's needs.

In the next sections, we will discuss some signs you need to watch out for that might indicate a need for dietary adjustments and how to safely introduce these changes to your dog's meals.

B. Identifying Signs of Nutritional Deficiencies

While a well-balanced homemade diet can provide all the necessary nutrients for your dog, sometimes, nutritional deficiencies may occur. It's important to recognize the signs of potential deficiencies to promptly address them. Here are some signs to look out for:

Lackluster Coat and Skin Issues:

If your dog's coat has lost its shine or appears dry and brittle, or if their skin is excessively dry, itchy, or flaky, this could be a sign of deficiency in essential fatty acids or certain vitamins.

Lethargy or Decreased Activity:

A decrease in energy levels could indicate a deficiency in various nutrients. It could mean your dog isn't getting enough protein, certain vitamins, or it could be a sign of anemia, often caused by iron deficiency.

Digestive Issues:

Persistent diarrhea or constipation might mean a deficiency or imbalance in dietary fiber. However, these symptoms can also suggest other health issues, so it's important to consult your vet.

Poor Growth in Puppies:

Puppies that don't grow at an expected rate may be deficient in certain nutrients, including protein, vitamins, or minerals like calcium and phosphorus.

Weight Loss or Gain:

Unexplained weight loss could mean your dog isn't getting enough calories, while unexplained weight gain could indicate too many calories or a lack of necessary exercise.

Weakness or Muscle Wasting:

If your dog seems weak or you notice a loss of muscle mass, they may not be getting enough protein or certain other nutrients.

Behavioral Changes:

Changes in behavior, such as increased aggression or anxiety, can sometimes be related to nutritional deficiencies, but they can also be signs of various health issues.

Remember, these signs can often be subtle and can be indicators of numerous health issues, not just nutritional deficiencies. It's essential to consult with your vet if you notice any changes in your dog. If nutritional deficiencies are identified, your vet can help you adjust your dog's diet to ensure they're getting all the necessary nutrients.

In the next section, we will discuss how to adjust your dog's diet if necessary, and the importance of making these changes gradually.

C. Making Necessary Adjustments to Your Dog's Diet

Just as with people, a dog's nutritional needs can change over time due to various factors such as age, health condition, activity level, and even the changing seasons. Regular vet check-ups can help identify any necessary adjustments to your dog's diet. Once identified, it's important to implement these changes in a way that is safe and comfortable for your dog. Here are some guidelines:

Make Changes Gradually:

Sudden changes in a dog's diet can cause digestive upset. Therefore, any changes should be introduced gradually, over a week or two. Start by replacing a small amount of the old diet with the new one, and gradually increase the new diet's proportion.

Monitor Your Dog's Response:

Keep a close eye on your dog as you introduce dietary changes. Watch for any signs of digestive upset, changes in appetite, or changes in behavior. If you notice anything concerning, contact your vet.

Maintain Balance:

Remember, balance is key in a dog's diet. If you're increasing or decreasing one component of the diet, other adjustments may be necessary to keep the diet balanced. For example, if you increase the amount of protein in your dog's diet, you may need to decrease the amount of carbohydrates to keep the caloric intake the same.

Consider Supplements:

If your dog has specific nutritional deficiencies, supplements may be necessary. Always consult with your vet before adding any supplements to your dog's diet.

Re-evaluate Regularly:

Once changes have been made, continue to monitor your dog's response over the long term. Regular vet check-ups can help evaluate whether the dietary changes are working or if further adjustments are needed.

Remember, every dog is unique, and what works for one may not work for another. A diet that suits your dog's individual needs, coupled with regular vet check-ups, will help ensure your dog lives a long, healthy, and happy life. In the next chapter, we will delve into specific scenarios where dietary adjustments may be necessary and provide guidelines on how to manage these situations.

XI. Conclusion: The Journey Towards a Healthier Dog

A. Reiteration of the Benefits of Homemade Dog Food

As we wrap up this comprehensive guide, let's revisit the numerous benefits of homemade dog food to reaffirm why taking the time and effort to prepare meals for your furry friend can be so rewarding.

Control Over Ingredients:
Homemade dog food gives you full control over what your dog is eating. This means you can ensure high-quality ingredients and avoid fillers, additives, or low-quality proteins often found in some commercial dog foods.

Tailored Nutrition:
Every dog is unique. With homemade food, you can tailor your dog's diet to their specific needs, whether they're a puppy, a senior, an active adult, or have particular health conditions.

Promotes Health and Longevity:
A balanced, nutritious diet promotes overall health and longevity. It can improve your dog's skin and coat, enhance their immune system, maintain healthy digestion, and keep their weight in check.

Variety:
Dogs appreciate variety, too! With homemade food, you can offer a range of different foods and flavors, keeping mealtime interesting for your dog.

Cost-Effective:
While it may seem expensive initially, homemade dog food can be cost-effective in the long run, especially when considering potential savings on vet bills related to poor nutrition.

Bonding Time:
Preparing meals for your dog can be a special bonding activity, showing your dog how much you care.

Peace of Mind:
Knowing exactly what your dog is eating can provide significant peace of mind, especially during times when commercial dog food recalls occur.

Remember, transitioning to homemade dog food is a journey, not a sprint. It's about gradually making changes that improve your dog's health and happiness. As you've learned throughout this book, the key to a successful transition is knowledge, patience, and regular vet check-ups.

In the following sections, we will provide a summary of the essential points from each chapter as a quick reference guide, and we will conclude with some final words of advice and encouragement for your homemade dog food journey.

B. Encouragement for Continued Exploration and Experimentation

We hope that this book has provided you with a solid foundation for starting your journey towards providing homemade, nutritious meals for your dog. But this is just the beginning. The world of dog nutrition is vast and ever-evolving, and there is always more to learn and explore.

Remember that each dog is unique, with their own preferences, dietary needs, and health conditions. What works for one dog may not work for another. Hence, don't be afraid to experiment, always under the guidance of your vet, of course. Try different recipes, ingredients, and meal plans, and observe your dog's reactions to them.

Here are a few words of encouragement as you continue on this journey:

Patience is Key:
Transitioning to homemade dog food, figuring out what works best for your dog, can take time. Don't be discouraged if you face challenges along the way. Patience and consistency are key.

Stay Informed:
Stay abreast of the latest research in dog nutrition. New discoveries and advancements are being made regularly that can further enhance your dog's health and well-being.

Embrace the Journey:
Enjoy the process. Take pleasure in preparing meals for your dog, knowing that you're contributing positively to their health and happiness.

Celebrate Small Wins:
Celebrate the improvements you see in your dog's health and vitality. Whether it's a shinier coat, more energy, or a healthier weight, each small victory is proof that your efforts are paying off.

Remember, the goal is not perfection, but progress. Even small changes can have a significant impact on your dog's health over time. Your dog doesn't need a perfect diet—they need a balanced, lovingly prepared diet that suits their individual needs.

In the next and final section of this book, we will provide a summary of each chapter for quick reference. This guide will serve as a handy tool as you continue to navigate the world of homemade dog food.

C. Final Thoughts on the Impact of Diet on a Dog's Health and Longevity

As we draw to a close, we want to emphasize one last time the profound impact that diet can have on a dog's health and longevity. Just as in humans, the food that your dog consumes plays a crucial role in their overall health, wellness, and quality of life.

A balanced, nutritious diet can:

Boost the Immune System: The right mix of vitamins, minerals, and antioxidants can help enhance your dog's immune system, making them more resilient to various diseases and infections.

Promote Healthy Weight: A diet tailored to your dog's age, breed, size, and activity level can help maintain a healthy weight, preventing issues like obesity, which can lead to numerous other health problems.

Enhance Skin and Coat Health: Essential fatty acids and other nutrients can promote a shiny coat and healthy skin, reducing issues like dryness, itching, and flaking.

Support Digestive Health: Adequate dietary fiber and quality proteins can support a healthy digestive system, reducing issues like diarrhea, constipation, and gas.

Support Joint Health: Especially in older dogs, a diet rich in certain nutrients can support joint health, reducing the risk of issues like arthritis.

Promote Longevity: Ultimately, all of the above benefits contribute to a longer, healthier life for your dog.

Making the decision to prepare homemade dog food is making a commitment to your dog's health and happiness. It's a labor of love that can offer immense rewards in the form of your dog's improved health, increased vitality, and potentially extended lifespan.

We hope this book has provided you with the knowledge, resources, and confidence you need to embark on this journey. Remember, you're not alone. There's a whole community of pet parents out there who are on this same journey, and numerous resources available to support you.

Your dog is a part of your family, and just like with any family member, you want the best for them. By choosing to feed your dog a homemade diet, you're choosing to offer them the very best.

Thank you for taking the time to read this book and for taking this important step towards improving your dog's health and happiness. Good luck on your homemade dog food journey!

XII. Appendices

A. Sample 28 Days Meal Plans

The following are some sample weekly meal plans that you can use as a starting point for feeding your dog homemade meals. These plans are based on a healthy adult dog of a medium breed. Portion sizes, and specific nutritional needs may vary based on your dog's age, weight, breed, and health status, so always consult your vet for guidance.

Day 1:
- Breakfast: Peanut Butter and Banana Oats
- Lunch: Rice and Veggie Mix
- Dinner: Chicken and Sweet Potato Hash
- Treat: Peanut Butter and Honey Dog Biscuits

Day 2:
- Breakfast: Blueberry and Spinach Smoothie
- Lunch: Cottage Cheese and Fruit
- Dinner: Fish and Brown Rice
- Treat: Blueberry and Banana Dog Cookies

Day 3:
- Breakfast: Apple and Turkey Sausage
- Lunch: Chicken Stew with Veggies
- Dinner: Lamb and Barley Bowl
- Treat: Quinoa and Pumpkin Dog Treats

Day 4:
- Breakfast: Sardine Scramble
- Lunch: Turkey and Rice Mix
- Dinner: Beef and Quinoa Dinner
- Treat: Chicken and Carrot Dog Biscuits

Day 5:
- Breakfast: Pumpkin and Quinoa Porridge
- Lunch: Fish and Sweet Potato
- Dinner: Liver and Brown Rice
- Treat: Salmon and Sweet Potato Treats

Day 6:
- Breakfast: Yogurt and Mixed Berries
- Lunch: Turkey and Vegetable Mix
- Dinner: Venison and Sweet Potato Dinner
- Treat: Beet and Cheese Dog Treats

Day 7:
- Breakfast: Chicken and Vegetable Casserole
- Lunch: Pork and Apple Dinner
- Dinner: Rabbit and Barley Bowl
- Treat: Zucchini and Apple Bites

Day 8:
- Breakfast: Peanut Butter and Banana Oats
- Lunch: Chicken Stew with Veggies
- Dinner: Salmon and Peas Dinner
- Treat: Peanut Butter and Honey Dog Biscuits

Day 9:
- Breakfast: Blueberry and Spinach Smoothie
- Lunch: Turkey and Rice Mix
- Dinner: Pork and Apple Dinner
- Treat: Blueberry and Banana Dog Cookies

Day 10:
- Breakfast: Apple and Turkey Sausage
- Lunch: Fish and Sweet Potato
- Dinner: Chicken and Vegetable Casserole
- Treat: Quinoa and Pumpkin Dog Treats

Day 11:
- Breakfast: Sardine Scramble
- Lunch: Turkey and Vegetable Mix
- Dinner: Rabbit and Barley Bowl

- Treat: Chicken and Carrot Dog Biscuits

Day 12:
- Breakfast: Pumpkin and Quinoa Porridge
- Lunch: Rice and Veggie Mix
- Dinner: Liver and Brown Rice
- Treat: Salmon and Sweet Potato Treats

Day 13:
- Breakfast: Yogurt and Mixed Berries
- Lunch: Cottage Cheese and Fruit
- Dinner: Lamb and Barley Bowl
- Treat: Beet and Cheese Dog Treats

Day 14:
- Breakfast: Chicken and Sweet Potato Hash
- Lunch: Fish and Brown Rice
- Dinner: Venison and Sweet Potato Dinner
- Treat: Zucchini and Apple Bites

Day 15:
- Breakfast: Peanut Butter and Banana Oats
- Lunch: Chicken and Vegetable Casserole
- Dinner: Salmon and Peas Dinner
- Treat: Peanut Butter and Honey Dog Biscuits

Day 16:
- Breakfast: Blueberry and Spinach Smoothie
- Lunch: Rabbit and Barley Bowl
- Dinner: Pork and Apple Dinner
- Treat: Blueberry and Banana Dog Cookies

Day 17:
- Breakfast: Apple and Turkey Sausage
- Lunch: Turkey and Rice Mix
- Dinner: Lamb and Barley Bowl
- Treat: Quinoa and Pumpkin Dog Treats

Day 18:
- Breakfast: Sardine Scramble
- Lunch: Fish and Sweet Potato

- Dinner: Liver and Brown Rice
- Treat: Chicken and Carrot Dog Biscuits

Day 19:
- Breakfast: Pumpkin and Quinoa Porridge
- Lunch: Rice and Veggie Mix
- Dinner: Chicken and Vegetable Casserole
- Treat: Salmon and Sweet Potato Treats

Day 20:
- Breakfast: Yogurt and Mixed Berries
- Lunch: Cottage Cheese and Fruit
- Dinner: Rabbit and Barley Bowl
- Treat: Beet and Cheese Dog Treats

Day 21:
- Breakfast: Chicken and Sweet Potato Hash
- Lunch: Fish and Brown Rice
- Dinner: Venison and Sweet Potato Dinner
- Treat: Zucchini and Apple Bites

Day 22:
- Breakfast: Cottage Cheese and Fruit
- Lunch: Turkey and Rice Mix
- Dinner: Rabbit and Barley Bowl
- Treat: Salmon and Sweet Potato Treats

Day 23:
- Breakfast: Yogurt and Mixed Berries
- Lunch: Chicken and Sweet Potato Hash
- Dinner: Pork and Apple Dinner
- Treat: Peanut Butter and Honey Dog Biscuits

Day 24:
- Breakfast: Peanut Butter and Banana Oats
- Lunch: Fish and Brown Rice
- Dinner: Turkey and Vegetable Mix
- Treat: Quinoa and Pumpkin Dog Treats

Day 25:
- Breakfast: Apple and Turkey Sausage

- Lunch: Lamb and Barley Bowl
- Dinner: Chicken and Vegetable Casserole
- Treat: Chicken and Carrot Dog Biscuits

Day 26:
- Breakfast: Sardine Scramble
- Lunch: Chicken Stew with Veggies
- Dinner: Beef and Quinoa Dinner
- Treat: Blueberry and Banana Dog Cookies

Day 27:
- Breakfast: Pumpkin and Quinoa Porridge
- Lunch: Rice and Veggie Mix
- Dinner: Liver and Brown Rice
- Treat: Beet and Cheese Dog Treats

Day 28:
- Breakfast: Blueberry and Spinach Smoothie
- Lunch: Fish and Sweet Potato
- Dinner: Venison and Sweet Potato Dinner
- Treat: Zucchini and Apple Bites

B. Nutritional Content of Common Ingredients

Understanding the nutritional content of common ingredients can greatly help in crafting balanced meals for your dog. Here's a brief overview of the nutrition provided by some frequently used ingredients in homemade dog foods:

Protein Sources:

Chicken: A lean source of protein, chicken also provides essential vitamins like B3 (niacin), B6, and minerals such as selenium, phosphorus, and zinc.

Beef: An excellent source of high-quality protein, beef also contains essential vitamins and minerals, including B vitamins, zinc, and iron.

Salmon: High in omega-3 fatty acids, salmon is beneficial for your dog's skin and coat. It's also a good source of protein and vitamin D.

Turkey: A lean source of protein, turkey also provides essential nutrients such as selenium, vitamin B6, and niacin.

Carbohydrates:

Brown Rice: A complex carbohydrate that provides steady energy, brown rice also contains fiber, vitamins, and minerals like magnesium and selenium.

Sweet Potato: Rich in beta carotene, fiber, and vitamins A, C, and B6, sweet potatoes are a nutritious carb source.

Quinoa: A pseudo-grain that is high in protein and rich in essential amino acids, fiber, and various vitamins and minerals.

Oats: High in fiber, oats also contain vitamins, minerals, and antioxidant compounds. They are a great source of energy for your dog.

Vegetables:

Carrots: High in fiber and beta carotene, which is converted to vitamin A in your dog's body.

Peas: Provide good amounts of vitamins A, K, and B vitamins, as well as minerals like iron, zinc, and manganese.

Pumpkin: A great source of fiber, vitamin A, and other nutrients, pumpkin is particularly good for digestion.

Spinach: A nutrient-dense leafy green, spinach provides vitamins A, C, K, and B vitamins, as well as minerals like iron and calcium.

Fruits:

Apples: A good source of fiber and vitamin C, just be sure to remove the seeds and core.

Blueberries: High in antioxidants, fiber, and vitamin C.

Bananas: A good source of potassium and vitamins C and B6.

Pears: High in fiber and vitamin C, ensure to remove the core and seeds.

Remember, it's important to introduce new foods slowly and in moderation to avoid digestive upset. It's also essential to balance these ingredients appropriately to meet your dog's nutritional needs. Always consult with your vet or a pet nutrition expert to ensure your homemade dog meals are balanced and healthy.

As you can see, making your dog's food from scratch can be a fun and healthy way to spend time with your animal friend. Always make sure to talk to your vet to make sure the food you give your pet meets its needs. With love, care, and a little time in the kitchen, you can give your dog a well-balanced meal with lots of different tastes. Here's to home-cooked meals that make dogs happy and healthier, one dish at a time. Don't forget that the time and work you put into your dog's health are well worth it because a healthy dog is a happy dog. "Good luck cooking!

SCAN THE QR CODE

OR COPY AND PASTE THE URL:

https://qrco.de/beMsz6

Made in United States
Troutdale, OR
01/04/2024

16675935R00058